Navigating the Depths of Kidney Failure

Understanding, Coping, and Conquering the Challenges of Kidney Failure

ADOOH MARCEL

DEDICATION

This book is dedicated to God almighty and my entire family for their unwavering support, boundless encouragement, and profound love they have showered upon me throughout my life and in the course of writing this book. They are the beating heart of my existence, and I want the world to know just how profoundly I appreciate their presence in my journey. And I pray that the almighty God bless them all.

Contents

Navigating the Depths of Kidney Failure 1

INTRODUCTION 8

CHAPTER ONE 10

UNDERSTANDING KIDNEY FAILURE 10

CAUSES AND RISK FACTORS 10

RISK FACTORS FOR KIDNEY FAILURE: 11

STAGES OF KIDNEY FAILURE 12

SIGNS AND SYMPTOMS 13

CHAPTER TWO 16

MEDICAL PERSPECTIVES 16

DIAGNOSING KIDNEY FAILURE 16

TREATMENT   OPTIONS   (MEDICATIONS,

DIALYSIS, TRANSPLANT) 18

LIFESTYLE CHANGES FOR KIDNEY HEALTH20

CHAPTER THREE 23

EMOTIONAL AND PSYCHOLOGICAL IMPACT...23

COPING WITH DIAGNOSIS..................................23

NAVIGATING THE EMOTIONAL ROLLERCOASTER..25

SUPPORT SYSTEMS...27

CHAPTER FOUR..30

DIET AND NUTRITION IN KIDNEY FAILURE 30

IMPORTANCE OF DIET IN RENAL HEALTH....30

FOODS TO LIMIT OR AVOID 32

CREATING A KIDNEY-FRIENDLY MEAL PLAN
....34

SAMPLE KIDNEY-FRIENDLY MEAL PLAN: 36

CHAPTER FIVE 38

LIFE WITH DIALYSIS 38

UNDERSTANDING DIALYSIS 38

COPING WITH THE CHALLENGES OF REGULAR DIALYSIS 41

CHAPTER SIX 45

PREVENTING KIDNEY FAILURE 45

LIFESTYLE CHANGES FOR PREVENTION 45

MANAGING CHRONIC CONDITIONS 48

REGULAR HEALTH CHECKUPS 53

CHAPTER SEVEN 57

LIVING WITH A TRANSPLANTED KIDNEY 57

THE TRANSPLANT PROCESS 57

POST-TRANSPLANT CARE.....................................60

EMOTIONAL AND PHYSICAL RECOVERY 64

CHAPTER EIGHT 69

CONCLUSION...69

INTRODUCTION

Kidney failure, also known as renal failure, is a medical condition in which the kidneys are no longer able to function adequately. The kidneys play a crucial role in maintaining the body's overall health by filtering and removing waste products and excess fluids from the blood, regulating electrolyte balance, and producing hormones that help control blood pressure and stimulate the production of red blood cells.

There are two main types of kidney failure: acute and chronic.

1. **Acute Kidney Failure:**
   - This is a sudden and often reversible loss of kidney function that occurs over a short period, usually a few hours to a few days.
   - Common causes include severe infections, dehydration, blockages in the urinary tract, and certain medications or toxins.
2. **Chronic Kidney Failure:**
   - This is a gradual and irreversible loss of kidney function over an extended period, often spanning months or years.
   - Common causes include diabetes, high blood pressure (hypertension), chronic glomerulonephritis, and polycystic kidney disease.

Symptoms of Kidney Failure: The symptoms of kidney failure can vary depending on whether it is acute or chronic, but they may include:

- Fatigue and weakness
- Swelling in the legs, ankles, or feet
- Shortness of breath
- Increased or decreased urine output
- Nausea and vomiting
- Persistent itching

- High blood pressure
- Confusion

Diagnosis and Treatment: Diagnosis often involves blood tests to measure levels of waste products, electrolytes, and other substances in the blood. Imaging studies, such as ultrasound or CT scans, may also be used.

Treatment options depend on the type and severity of kidney failure. Acute kidney failure may be reversible with prompt treatment of the underlying cause, while chronic kidney failure may require ongoing management, including medications, dietary changes, and, in severe cases, dialysis or kidney transplantation.

Prevention: Preventing kidney failure involves managing risk factors such as controlling blood pressure, managing diabetes, staying hydrated, and avoiding exposure to toxins and medications that can harm the kidneys.

It's crucial for individuals at risk or experiencing symptoms of kidney failure to seek medical attention promptly. Early detection and intervention can significantly improve outcomes and quality of life for those affected by kidney failure.

CHAPTER ONE
UNDERSTANDING KIDNEY FAILURE

Understanding kidney failure involves exploring the causes, symptoms, diagnosis, and treatment options associated with this condition. Let's delve deeper into these aspects:

CAUSES AND RISK FACTORS

Kidney failure can be caused by a variety of factors, and certain individuals are at a higher risk of developing this condition. Here are some common causes and risk factors associated with kidney failure:

CAUSES OF KIDNEY FAILURE:

1. **Chronic Diseases:**
    - **Diabetes:** Uncontrolled diabetes is a leading cause of kidney failure. High blood sugar levels can damage the small blood vessels in the kidneys over time, affecting their function.
    - **Hypertension (High Blood Pressure):** Prolonged high blood pressure can strain and damage the blood vessels in the kidneys, leading to kidney failure.
    - **Chronic Glomerulonephritis:** Inflammation of the glomeruli, the kidney's filtering units, can result in kidney damage over time.
2. **Acute Conditions:**
    - **Infections:** Severe infections, especially those affecting the urinary tract, can lead to acute kidney failure.
    - **Dehydration:** Insufficient fluid intake can lead to a decrease in blood volume, affecting kidney function.
    - **Obstruction:** Blockages in the urinary tract, such as kidney stones or tumors, can impede the flow of urine and lead to kidney damage.
3. **Other Causes:**

- **Polycystic Kidney Disease (PKD):** A genetic disorder where fluid-filled cysts develop in the kidneys, gradually replacing normal tissue and impairing kidney function.
- **Autoimmune Diseases:** Conditions like lupus and certain immune system disorders can affect the kidneys.
- **Medications and Toxins:** Some drugs, over-the-counter medications, and toxins can cause kidney damage if taken in excess or over an extended period.
- **Trauma:** Severe physical injury or trauma to the kidneys can lead to kidney failure.

RISK FACTORS FOR KIDNEY FAILURE:

1. **Age:** The risk of kidney failure tends to increase with age.
2. **Family History:** A family history of kidney disease, especially genetic conditions like PKD, can increase the risk.
3. **Race and Ethnicity:** Some ethnic groups, such as African Americans, Hispanics, and Native Americans, have a higher risk of developing kidney disease.
4. **Gender:** Men are generally at a higher risk of kidney failure than women.
5. **Genetics:** Certain genetic factors may predispose individuals to kidney diseases.
6. **Obesity:** Being overweight or obese is associated with an increased risk of kidney disease.
7. **Smoking:** Smoking can contribute to the progression of kidney disease.
8. **Cardiovascular Disease:** Conditions such as heart disease and atherosclerosis can impact kidney function.
9. **Certain Medical Conditions:** Conditions like systemic lupus erythematosus (lupus) and multiple myeloma can increase the risk of kidney disease.

It's important to note that some risk factors can be modified through lifestyle changes and medical management. Regular health check-ups, monitoring of blood pressure and blood sugar levels, and adopting a healthy lifestyle can contribute to the prevention or early detection of kidney disease. If individuals have one or more risk factors, they should work closely with healthcare professionals to manage their overall health and reduce the risk of kidney failure.

STAGES OF KIDNEY FAILURE

Kidney failure, also known as renal failure, is typically classified into different stages based on the severity of impairment in kidney function. The commonly used system to categorize these stages is the Glomerular Filtration Rate (GFR), which is a measure of how efficiently the kidneys are filtering waste from the blood. The stages are as follows:

1. **Stage 1: Kidney Damage with Normal or Increased GFR (GFR > 90 ml/min):**
   - In this early stage, there is kidney damage, but the GFR is still normal or may be higher than normal. There may be other signs of kidney damage, such as the presence of protein in the urine.
2. **Stage 2: Mildly Decreased GFR (GFR = 60-89 ml/min):**
   - Kidney function is mildly reduced, but the kidneys can still effectively filter waste products from the blood. Like in Stage 1, there may be evidence of kidney damage, such as protein in the urine.
3. **Stage 3: Moderately Decreased GFR (GFR = 30-59 ml/min):**
   - This stage is further divided into Stage 3a (GFR = 45-59 ml/min) and Stage 3b (GFR = 30-44 ml/min). At this point, there is a noticeable decrease in kidney function, and individuals may start experiencing symptoms like fatigue and swelling.
4. **Stage 4: Severely Decreased GFR (GFR = 15-29 ml/min):**
   - Stage 4 is divided into Stage 4a (GFR = 15-29 ml/min) and Stage 4b (GFR < 15 ml/min). Kidney function is significantly reduced, and individuals may experience more pronounced symptoms. At this stage, discussions about

kidney replacement therapy options, such as dialysis or transplantation, often begin.

5. **Stage 5: End-Stage Kidney Disease (GFR < 15 ml/min):**
   - Also known as end-stage renal disease (ESRD), this is the final stage of kidney failure. GFR is very low, and kidney function is severely impaired. Individuals in Stage 5 typically require kidney replacement therapy, such as dialysis or kidney transplantation, to sustain life.

It's important to note that the progression through these stages can vary from person to person, and not everyone with kidney damage progresses to end-stage kidney disease. Some underlying causes of kidney disease may be reversible or manageable, especially if detected in the earlier stages.

Monitoring kidney function through regular check-ups, blood tests, and urine tests is crucial for the early detection and management of kidney disease. Lifestyle modifications, medications, and other interventions can help slow down the progression of kidney disease and improve overall outcomes. Individuals at risk or with kidney disease should work closely with healthcare professionals to develop a personalized treatment plan.

SIGNS AND SYMPTOMS

The signs and symptoms of kidney failure can vary depending on the underlying cause, the stage of kidney disease, and individual factors. In the early stages, kidney disease may not present noticeable symptoms. As the condition progresses, however, the following signs and symptoms may become more apparent:

1. **Changes in Urination:**
   - Changes in the frequency of urination.
   - Changes in the color and appearance of urine.
   - Difficulty or pain during urination.
   - Foamy or bubbly urine.
2. **Swelling:**

- Swelling in the face, hands, legs, ankles, or feet (edema). This is due to the kidneys' inability to effectively remove excess fluid from the body.

3. **Fatigue and Weakness:**
   - Feeling unusually tired or weak, even after getting enough rest.

4. **Shortness of Breath:**
   - Difficulty breathing or shortness of breath, often due to fluid buildup in the lungs.

5. **Itching:**
   - Persistent itching, often accompanied by dry skin. This can result from the buildup of waste products in the blood.

6. **Nausea and Vomiting:**
   - Feeling nauseous and experiencing vomiting, this may be related to the accumulation of waste products in the body.

7. **Loss of Appetite:**
   - A decrease in appetite or a metallic taste in the mouth.

8. **Hypertension (High Blood Pressure):**
   - Elevated blood pressure, which can be both a cause and a consequence of kidney disease.

9. **Muscle Cramps and Twitching:**
   - Muscle cramps, twitches, or weakness, which may be related to electrolyte imbalances.

10. **Difficulty Concentrating:**
    - Mental fogginess, difficulty concentrating, or memory issues.

11. **Sleep Problems:**
    - Difficulty sleeping or restless leg syndrome, which can be associated with kidney dysfunction.

12. **Puffiness Around the Eyes:**
    - Swelling or puffiness around the eyes, especially in the morning.

It's crucial to note that these symptoms can also be associated with other medical conditions and experiencing one or more of them does not necessarily mean a person has kidney failure. However, if individuals notice persistent or worsening symptoms, especially if they have risk factors for kidney disease, it's important to seek medical attention promptly.

Early detection of kidney disease allows for interventions that can slow or halt its progression. Regular check-ups, blood pressure monitoring, and kidney function tests are essential for individuals at risk of kidney disease or those with existing kidney conditions.

CHAPTER TWO
MEDICAL PERSPECTIVES

From a medical perspective, the evaluation and management of kidney failure involve various diagnostic tools, treatment strategies, and considerations. Here are some key medical perspectives on kidney failure:

DIAGNOSING KIDNEY FAILURE

Diagnosing kidney failure involves a combination of clinical evaluation, laboratory tests, and imaging studies. Here are the key steps and diagnostic tools commonly used in the diagnosis of kidney failure:

1. Medical History and Physical Examination:

- A thorough medical history is taken to identify risk factors, symptoms, and potential causes of kidney disease.
- A physical examination may reveal signs such as swelling, elevated blood pressure, or other indications of kidney dysfunction.

2. Blood Tests:

- **Serum Creatinine:** Elevated levels of creatinine in the blood indicate impaired kidney function. Creatinine is a waste product that the kidneys normally filter out.
- **Blood Urea Nitrogen (BUN):** Elevated BUN levels can suggest impaired kidney function, although it is less specific than creatinine.
- **Electrolyte Levels:** Abnormal levels of electrolytes, such as potassium and calcium, can be indicative of kidney dysfunction.

3. Glomerular Filtration Rate (GFR):

- GFR is a calculated value that estimates the kidneys' filtering capacity. It is determined based on serum creatinine levels, age, sex, and other factors.
- A GFR below normal levels indicates decreased kidney function, and the stage of kidney disease is classified based on the GFR.

4. Urinalysis:

- A urine sample is analyzed to check for the presence of abnormalities, such as protein, blood, or white blood cells.
- Abnormalities in the urine can provide clues about the underlying cause of kidney dysfunction.

5. Imaging Studies:

- **Ultrasound:** This imaging technique provides detailed images of the kidneys and can help identify structural abnormalities, cysts, or obstructions.
- **CT scan or MRI:** These imaging studies may be used for more detailed visualization of the kidneys and surrounding structures, especially in cases where ultrasound results are inconclusive.

6. Kidney Biopsy:

- In certain cases, a kidney biopsy may be performed to obtain a small tissue sample for microscopic examination. This is typically done when the cause of kidney disease is unclear or if a more detailed analysis is needed to guide treatment.

7. Additional Tests:

- Additional tests may be conducted based on the suspected cause of kidney failure. For example, tests for autoimmune disorders, infections, or specific kidney diseases may be ordered.

It's important to note that the diagnosis of kidney failure is often a process that involves assessing multiple factors and considering the patient's overall health. Early detection is crucial for implementing interventions that can slow or halt the progression of kidney disease. Individuals at risk, such as those with diabetes, hypertension, or a family history of kidney disease, should undergo regular screenings to monitor kidney function. If kidney disease is suspected or confirmed, a healthcare professional, often a nephrologist (a kidney specialist), will work with the patient to develop an appropriate treatment plan.

TREATMENT OPTIONS (MEDICATIONS, DIALYSIS, TRANSPLANT)

The treatment options for kidney failure depend on the underlying cause, the severity of the condition, and individual factors. Here are the main treatment modalities for kidney failure:

1. **Medications:**
   - **Blood Pressure Medications:** Controlling blood pressure is crucial in managing kidney failure. Medications such as angiotensin-converting enzyme (ACE) inhibitors or angiotensin II receptor blockers (ARBs) are commonly prescribed.
   - **Diuretics:** These medications help eliminate excess fluid from the body, reducing swelling and managing fluid balance.
   - **Erythropoiesis-Stimulating Agents (ESAs):** In cases of anemia associated with kidney failure, ESAs may be prescribed to stimulate the production of red blood cells.

- **Phosphate Binders and Vitamin D:** These medications help manage imbalances in phosphorus and calcium levels in the blood.

2. **Dietary Changes:**
   - A controlled diet may be recommended to manage symptoms and slow the progression of kidney disease. This often includes restrictions on sodium, potassium, and phosphorus intake.

3. **Dialysis:**
   - **Hemodialysis:** This process involves using a machine to filter and clean the blood. It is typically performed at a dialysis center, and sessions are usually scheduled several times a week.
   - **Peritoneal Dialysis:** This type of dialysis involves using the lining of the abdomen (peritoneum) as a natural filter. It can be done at home, offering more flexibility in treatment.

4. **Kidney Transplant:**
   - A kidney transplant is a surgical procedure in which a healthy kidney from a living or deceased donor is transplanted into a person with kidney failure.
   - Transplantation offers the potential for a more normal and active life, with fewer dietary restrictions and a reduced need for ongoing medical interventions.

5. **Management of Underlying Causes:**
   - Identifying and managing the underlying causes of kidney failure is essential. This may involve treating conditions such as diabetes, hypertension, or autoimmune disorders.

6. **Symptomatic Treatment:**
   - Depending on the symptoms and complications of kidney failure, additional medications or interventions may be prescribed to manage specific issues. For example, medications to control itching or to address metabolic acidosis may be used.

It's important to note that the choice of treatment depends on factors such as the patient's overall health, lifestyle, preferences, and the availability of resources. The decision on the most appropriate treatment plan is typically made in collaboration between the patient and a healthcare team, which may include nephrologists, dietitians, and other specialists.

Regular monitoring and follow-up care are essential for individuals with kidney failure to adjust treatment plans as needed and manage potential complications. The goal of treatment is to improve the quality of life, manage symptoms, and slow the progression of kidney disease.

LIFESTYLE CHANGES FOR KIDNEY HEALTH

Adopting a healthy lifestyle is crucial for maintaining kidney health and preventing or managing kidney disease. Here are some key lifestyle changes that can support kidney health:

1. **Stay Hydrated:**
   - Drinking an adequate amount of water is essential for kidney function. It helps flush out toxins and waste products from the body.
2. **Balanced Diet:**
   - Follow a well-balanced diet that includes a variety of fruits, vegetables, whole grains, lean proteins, and limited amounts of saturated and trans fats.
   - Manage portion sizes and be mindful of your salt intake. High sodium levels can contribute to high blood pressure, which is a risk factor for kidney disease.
3. **Limit Processed Foods:**
   - Processed and packaged foods often contain high levels of sodium, phosphorus, and other additives that can be harmful to kidney health. Choose fresh, whole foods whenever possible.
4. **Control Blood Sugar Levels:**
   - If you have diabetes, it's crucial to manage blood sugar levels through medication, diet, and regular monitoring. Elevated blood sugar can contribute to kidney damage.

5. **Control Blood Pressure:**
   - High blood pressure is a leading cause of kidney disease. Regular exercise, a healthy diet, and medications prescribed by your healthcare provider can help manage blood pressure.
6. **Maintain a Healthy Weight:**
   - Being overweight or obese increases the risk of kidney disease. Adopting a healthy diet and engaging in regular physical activity can help achieve and maintain a healthy weight.
7. **Exercise Regularly:**
   - Regular physical activity improves overall cardiovascular health and can help control conditions such as diabetes and hypertension, which are risk factors for kidney disease.
8. **Avoid Excessive Use of NSAIDs:**
   - Nonsteroidal anti-inflammatory drugs (NSAIDs), such as ibuprofen and naproxen, can cause kidney damage if used excessively. Consult with your healthcare provider about alternative pain management options.
9. **Limit Alcohol Intake:**
   - Excessive alcohol consumption can contribute to high blood pressure and other health problems. Limit alcohol intake to moderate levels or as advised by your healthcare provider.
10. **Quit Smoking:**
    - Smoking can worsen kidney function and is a risk factor for kidney disease. Quitting smoking improves overall health and reduces the risk of kidney damage.
11. **Manage Stress:**
    - Chronic stress can contribute to health problems, including hypertension. Practice stress-reducing activities such as meditation, yoga, or deep breathing exercises.
12. **Get Regular Check-ups:**
    - Regular health check-ups, including monitoring blood pressure, blood sugar, and kidney function, can help detect and manage potential issues early on.

It's important to note that these lifestyle changes are beneficial not only for kidney health but for overall well-being. If you have specific concerns about your kidney health or if you have risk factors for kidney disease, consult with a healthcare professional for personalized advice and guidance.

CHAPTER THREE
EMOTIONAL AND PSYCHOLOGICAL IMPACT

The diagnosis and management of kidney failure can have a profound emotional and psychological impact on individuals and their families. Coping with the challenges associated with kidney failure involves addressing various aspects of emotional well-being. Here are some key considerations:

COPING WITH DIAGNOSIS

Coping with a diagnosis of kidney failure can be challenging, but there are various strategies and resources available to help individuals and their families navigate this journey. Here are some coping strategies:

1. **Educate Yourself:**
   - Understanding the nature of kidney failure, available treatments, and lifestyle modifications can empower you to actively participate in your care. Ask your healthcare team for information and resources.
2. **Build a Support System:**
   - Share your feelings with trusted friends, family members, or support groups. A strong support system can provide emotional support, understanding, and practical assistance.
3. **Communicate Openly:**
   - Keep open lines of communication with your healthcare team. Discuss your concerns, ask questions, and actively participate in decision-making about your treatment plan.
4. **Seek Professional Counseling:**
   - Mental health professionals, such as counselors or psychologists, can provide valuable support in coping with the emotional impact of kidney failure. They can help you

develop coping strategies and provide a safe space to express your feelings.

5. **Join Support Groups:**
   - Connecting with others who are going through similar experiences can be reassuring and provide a sense of community. Many local and online support groups cater to individuals with kidney disease and their families.

6. **Set Realistic Goals:**
   - Break down large tasks into smaller, manageable goals. Setting realistic and achievable goals can help maintain a sense of control and accomplishment.

7. **Maintain a Positive Outlook:**
   - Focus on aspects of your life that bring joy and positivity. Cultivate gratitude and celebrate small victories. A positive mindset can contribute to overall well-being.

8. **Explore Stress-Relief Techniques:**
   - Incorporate stress-relief techniques into your daily routine, such as meditation, deep breathing exercises, yoga, or mindfulness. These practices can help manage anxiety and improve mental well-being.

9. **Balance Emotional Expression:**
   - It's okay to express a range of emotions, including sadness, anger, or frustration. Allow yourself time to grieve and process the impact of the diagnosis.

10. **Maintain Physical Health:**
    - Stay physically active within the limits of your condition. Regular exercise can contribute to both physical and mental well-being.

11. **Adapt to Lifestyle Changes:**
    - Embrace necessary lifestyle changes, including dietary modifications and treatment plans. Collaborate with your healthcare team to find strategies that work for you.

12. **Address Financial Concerns:**
    - If you have financial concerns related to the cost of medical care, medications, or lifestyle changes, seek guidance from financial counselors and explore available resources.

13. **Involve Loved Ones:**
    - Include family members and loved ones in discussions about your condition and treatment. Their support can be invaluable, and involving them in the process fosters a sense of shared responsibility.

Remember that coping with a chronic condition is a process, and it's okay to seek help when needed. Each person's experience is unique, and finding a personalized approach to coping is essential. If you find yourself struggling, don't hesitate to reach out to your healthcare team for additional support and guidance.

NAVIGATING THE EMOTIONAL ROLLERCOASTER

Navigating the emotional rollercoaster associated with a diagnosis of kidney failure requires resilience, self-awareness, and ongoing support. Here are some strategies to help manage the emotional ups and downs:

1. **Acknowledge and Validate Emotions:**
   - Understand that it's normal to experience a range of emotions, including fear, anger, sadness, and even moments of hope. Acknowledge these feelings without judgment.
2. **Seek Professional Support:**
   - Consider talking to a mental health professional, such as a counselor or psychologist, who can provide guidance, coping strategies, and a safe space to express your emotions.
3. **Maintain Open Communication:**
   - Keep the lines of communication open with your healthcare team, friends, and family. Share your thoughts, concerns, and feelings with those you trust.
4. **Join Support Groups:**
   - Connect with others who are facing similar challenges through support groups. Sharing experiences with individuals who understand can provide a sense of community and validation.

5. **Practice Mindfulness and Relaxation Techniques:**
   - Engage in mindfulness practices, meditation, deep breathing exercises, or progressive muscle relaxation to help manage stress and promote emotional well-being.
6. **Set Realistic Expectations:**
   - Recognize that adapting to the changes associated with kidney failure is a gradual process. Set realistic expectations for yourself and celebrate small victories along the way.
7. **Focus on What You Can Control:**
   - Identify aspects of your life that you can control and take steps to manage them. This may include following your treatment plan, making healthy lifestyle choices, and maintaining a positive mindset.
8. **Involve Loved Ones:**
   - Share your experiences and concerns with family members and loved ones. Their support can provide comfort and assistance in navigating challenges.
9. **Celebrate Positivity:**
   - Cultivate gratitude by focusing on positive aspects of your life. Celebrate moments of joy, progress, and resilience.
10. **Adapt and Embrace Change:**
    - Acknowledge that living with kidney failure may involve lifestyle changes. Embrace these changes as part of your journey and focus on the aspects you can control.
11. **Stay Informed:**
    - Educate yourself about your condition and treatment options. Understanding the medical aspects can empower you and reduce anxiety about the unknown.
12. **Balance Emotional Expression:**
    - Allow yourself to express a range of emotions. Share your feelings with others or express them through creative outlets like writing or art.
13. **Take Breaks and Practice Self-Care:**
    - Give yourself permission to take breaks when needed. Engage in activities that bring you joy and relaxation,

whether it's reading, listening to music, or spending time in nature.

14. **Plan for the Future:**
    - While focusing on the present, it can be helpful to plan for the future. This may include discussing long-term goals, aspirations, and potential adjustments to your lifestyle.

Remember that emotional well-being is an ongoing process, and it's okay to seek support when needed. Building a support network, both within the healthcare system and through personal connections, is crucial for navigating the emotional challenges associated with kidney failure.

SUPPORT SYSTEMS

Building a strong support system is crucial for individuals facing kidney failure. This network can provide emotional, practical, and informational support, helping individuals navigate the challenges associated with their condition. Here are key elements of a supportive network:

1. **Family and Friends:**
    - **Emotional Support:** Loved ones can offer understanding, empathy, and a listening ear during difficult times.
    - **Practical Support:** Family and friends can assist with daily tasks, transportation to medical appointments, and other practical needs.
2. **Healthcare Team:**
    - **Nephrologists and Healthcare Professionals:** Your medical team plays a central role in your care. Establish open communication with your nephrologist and other healthcare professionals to discuss your concerns and receive guidance.
3. **Support Groups:**
    - Joining support groups for individuals with kidney disease or chronic illnesses allows you to connect with others who share similar experiences. These groups can provide a sense of community, understanding, and valuable insights.

4. **Mental Health Professionals:**
   - **Counselors or Psychologists:** Mental health professionals can offer emotional support, coping strategies, and a safe space to discuss the emotional impact of kidney failure.
5. **Dietitians and Nutritionists:**
   - **Dietary Support:** Working with a dietitian or nutritionist can help you navigate dietary restrictions and create meal plans that align with your health needs.
6. **Financial Counselors:**
   - **Financial Support:** If you have concerns about the financial aspects of managing kidney failure, financial counselors can provide guidance on available resources, insurance coverage, and financial planning.
7. **Caregivers:**
   - If you have a caregiver, ensure they are well-informed about your condition and treatment plan. They can provide invaluable support in managing daily tasks, attending medical appointments, and offering emotional support.
8. **Spiritual or Religious Support:**
   - If spirituality or religion is important to you, seek support from your faith community. Spiritual leaders and community members can offer comfort, guidance, and a sense of purpose.
9. **Patient Advocacy Organizations:**
   - Organizations dedicated to kidney health can provide informational resources, educational materials, and advocacy support. They may also offer events or programs that connect individuals facing similar challenges.
10. **Online Communities:**
    - Participating in online forums or communities related to kidney health allows you to connect with a broader network of individuals. These platforms provide a space for sharing experiences and exchanging information.
11. **Educational Resources:**
    - Stay informed about your condition and treatment options through reputable educational resources. Knowledge

empowers you to actively participate in your care and make informed decisions.

12. **Employer and Workplace Support:**
    - Communicate with your employer about your condition and explore available workplace accommodations. A supportive work environment can contribute to overall well-being.

Building and maintaining a support system is an ongoing process. Regular communication, both with healthcare professionals and personal connections, is essential. Remember that everyone's support needs are unique, so tailor your network to meet your specific emotional, practical, and informational needs as you navigate kidney failure.

CHAPTER FOUR
DIET AND NUTRITION IN KIDNEY FAILURE

Diet and nutrition play a crucial role in managing kidney failure. Individuals with kidney failure often need to make specific dietary adjustments to support overall health and manage symptoms. Here are key considerations for diet and nutrition in kidney failure:

IMPORTANCE OF DIET IN RENAL HEALTH

Diet plays a fundamental role in maintaining renal health, and it becomes especially crucial in preventing and managing kidney disease. Here are key reasons highlighting the importance of diet in renal health:

1. **Managing Blood Pressure:**
   - **Role:** Hypertension (high blood pressure) is a leading cause of kidney disease. A diet low in sodium and rich in potassium, as well as other heart-healthy nutrients, helps regulate blood pressure and protects kidney function.
2. **Controlling Blood Sugar Levels:**
   - **Role:** For individuals with diabetes, uncontrolled blood sugar levels can contribute to kidney damage. A well-balanced diet that manages carbohydrate intake and emphasizes whole foods is essential in diabetes management and kidney protection.
3. **Reducing Protein Intake in Kidney Disease:**
   - **Role:** In chronic kidney disease (CKD), reducing the intake of protein can alleviate the workload on the kidneys, which may be impaired in their ability to excrete waste products efficiently.
4. **Minimizing Phosphorus and Potassium Intake:**
   - **Role:** Impaired kidneys may struggle to regulate phosphorus and potassium levels in the blood. Restricting the intake of

foods high in these minerals can help prevent complications associated with imbalances.

5. **Preventing Fluid Overload:**
   - **Role:** Limiting fluid intake, including water and beverages, is crucial in preventing fluid overload in individuals with advanced kidney disease. This helps manage conditions like edema and hypertension.

6. **Supporting Overall Nutritional Health:**
   - **Role:** A balanced and nutrient-rich diet supports overall health, including maintaining a healthy weight, providing energy, and supplying essential vitamins and minerals necessary for various bodily functions.

7. **Managing Acid-Base Balance:**
   - **Role:** Kidneys play a crucial role in maintaining the body's acid-base balance. Certain dietary choices can impact this balance, and a well-designed diet helps support kidney function in this aspect.

8. **Reducing Oxidative Stress and Inflammation:**
   - **Role:** Chronic kidney disease is associated with oxidative stress and inflammation. Antioxidant-rich foods, such as fruits and vegetables, can help mitigate these factors.

9. **Delaying Progression of Kidney Disease:**
   - **Role:** Adhering to a kidney-friendly diet, along with other lifestyle modifications, can slow down the progression of kidney disease and delay the onset of end-stage renal disease.

10. **Preventing Malnutrition:**
    - **Role:** Individuals with kidney disease are at risk of malnutrition due to dietary restrictions and the body's increased nutrient needs. A carefully planned diet helps prevent malnutrition and supports optimal health.

11. **Improving Quality of Life:**
    - **Role:** Adapting the diet to individual needs and preferences contributes to an improved quality of life for individuals with kidney disease. This includes managing symptoms, maintaining energy levels, and supporting overall well-being.

12.

13. **Integrating with Medical Treatment:**
    - **Role:** Diet is an integral part of the comprehensive treatment plan for kidney disease. It works synergistically with medications and other medical interventions to optimize health outcomes.

It's important to note that dietary recommendations may vary based on the stage of kidney disease, individual health status, and the presence of other medical conditions. Therefore, individuals with kidney disease should work closely with a registered dietitian or nutritionist specializing in renal health to create a personalized and effective dietary plan.

FOODS TO LIMIT OR AVOID

For individuals with kidney disease, especially those in advanced stages, certain foods may need to be limited or avoided to help manage the condition and prevent complications. Here are some foods that are often restricted in a kidney-friendly diet:

1. **High-Sodium Foods:**
    - **Reason:** Sodium can contribute to fluid retention and elevated blood pressure, which are common concerns in kidney disease.
    - **Foods to Limit or Avoid:** Processed and packaged foods, canned soups, salty snacks, fast food, and restaurant-prepared dishes.
2. **High-Potassium Foods:**
    - **Reason:** Impaired kidneys may struggle to regulate potassium levels, leading to the risk of hyperkalemia (high potassium levels).
    - **Foods to Limit or Avoid:** Bananas, oranges, tomatoes, potatoes, sweet potatoes, spinach, avocados, and high-potassium salt substitutes.

3. **High-Phosphorus Foods:**
   - **Reason:** Kidneys with reduced function may have difficulty eliminating excess phosphorus, leading to imbalances in the body.
   - **Foods to Limit or Avoid:** Dairy products, nuts, seeds, chocolate, processed meats, and certain carbonated beverages.
4. **High-Protein Foods:**
   - **Reason:** Excessive protein intake can increase the workload on the kidneys, particularly in advanced stages of kidney disease.
   - **Foods to Limit or Avoid:** Red meat, poultry, fish, eggs, dairy products, and protein supplements.
5. **Processed and Fast Foods:**
   - **Reason:** These foods often contain high levels of sodium, phosphorus additives, and unhealthy fats, contributing to various complications in kidney disease.
   - **Foods to Limit or Avoid:** Fast food, frozen meals, processed snacks, and convenience foods.
6. **Dark-Colored Sodas:**
   - **Reason:** Dark sodas may contain phosphoric acid, which can contribute to increased phosphorus levels.
   - **Foods to Limit or Avoid:** Colas and other dark-colored sodas.
7. **Certain Fruits and Vegetables:**
   - **Reason:** While fruits and vegetables are generally healthy, some may be high in potassium.
   - **Foods to Limit or Avoid:** Oranges, bananas, tomatoes, potatoes, spinach, and avocados.
8. **Certain Whole Grains:**
   - **Reason:** Whole grains may contain more phosphorus compared to refined grains.
   - **Foods to Limit or Avoid:** Whole wheat, bran, and whole grain cereals.

9. **Dairy Products:**
    - **Reason:** Dairy products are a significant source of phosphorus and potassium.
    - **Foods to Limit or Avoid:** Milk, cheese, yogurt, and other dairy items.
10. **High-Sugar Foods:**
    - **Reason:** Diabetes is a common cause of kidney disease, and managing blood sugar levels is crucial.
    - **Foods to Limit or Avoid:** Candies, sugary beverages, desserts, and other high-sugar foods.

It's important to note that dietary restrictions can vary based on individual health conditions, the stage of kidney disease, and other factors. Consultation with a registered dietitian or nutritionist specializing in kidney health is crucial to creating a personalized dietary plan that meets nutritional needs while managing the specific challenges of kidney disease.

CREATING A KIDNEY-FRIENDLY MEAL PLAN

Creating a kidney-friendly meal plan involves careful consideration of nutrient intake to support overall health while managing specific dietary restrictions associated with kidney disease. Here are general guidelines for creating a kidney-friendly meal plan:

PROTEIN INTAKE:

1. **Choose High-Quality Proteins:**
    - Opt for lean protein sources such as skinless poultry, fish, eggs, and plant-based proteins like beans and tofu.
    - Limit red meat and processed meats, which tend to be higher in phosphorus and saturated fats.
2. **Control Portion Sizes:**
    - Moderation is key. Be mindful of portion sizes to avoid excessive protein intake.

PHOSPHORUS MANAGEMENT:

3. **Limit Phosphorus-Rich Foods:**
   - Reduce intake of dairy products, nuts, seeds, chocolate, and whole grains.
   - Choose low-phosphorus alternatives, such as rice milk or almond milk.

POTASSIUM MANAGEMENT:

4. **Choose Low-Potassium Fruits and Vegetables:**
   - Opt for fruits and vegetables with lower potassium content, such as apples, berries, and green beans.
   - Remove or leach high-potassium vegetables like potatoes to reduce potassium content.

SODIUM CONTROL:

5. **Reduce Sodium Intake:**
   - Choose fresh, whole foods over processed and packaged options.
   - Use herbs, spices, and lemon juice for flavoring instead of salt.
   - Rinse canned vegetables and beans to lower sodium content.

FLUID MANAGEMENT:

6. **Monitor Fluid Intake:**
   - Follow your healthcare provider's guidelines for daily fluid limits.
   - Spread fluid intake throughout the day and be mindful of beverages with added sugars.

SAMPLE KIDNEY-FRIENDLY MEAL PLAN:

BREAKFAST:

- **Option 1:** Oatmeal made with water, topped with sliced apples and a sprinkle of cinnamon.
- **Option 2:** Scrambled eggs with spinach and tomatoes.

SNACK:

- **Option 1:** Fresh berries.
- **Option 2:** Greek yogurt (portion-controlled).

LUNCH:

- **Option 1:** Grilled chicken salad with mixed greens, cucumber, and a vinaigrette dressing.
- **Option 2:** Quinoa salad with diced vegetables and chickpeas.

SNACK:

- **Option 1:** Carrot sticks with hummus.
- **Option 2:** Air-popped popcorn.

DINNER:

- **Option 1:** Baked or grilled fish with steamed asparagus and quinoa.
- **Option 2:** Stir-fried tofu with broccoli and brown rice.

DESSERT (IN MODERATION):

- **Option 1:** Fresh fruit salad.
- **Option 2:** Sorbet or sherbet.

GENERAL TIPS:

- **Work with a Dietitian:** A registered dietitian specializing in renal nutrition can tailor a meal plan to your specific needs.
- **Monitor Nutrient Levels:** Regularly monitor blood levels of phosphorus, potassium, and other relevant markers.
- **Individualized Approach:** Adjust the meal plan based on your specific dietary restrictions, preferences, and health goals.

Remember, this is a general guide, and individual needs may vary. It's essential to consult with a healthcare professional or dietitian to create a personalized meal plan that meets your specific requirements and supports your overall well-being.

CHAPTER FIVE
LIFE WITH DIALYSIS

Living with dialysis is a significant lifestyle adjustment for individuals with kidney failure. Dialysis is a life-sustaining treatment that helps perform the functions of the kidneys when they are no longer able to do so. Here are key aspects of life with dialysis:

UNDERSTANDING DIALYSIS

Dialysis is a medical procedure used to replicate some of the functions of the kidneys when they are no longer able to function properly. There are two main types of dialysis: hemodialysis and peritoneal dialysis.

1. HEMODIALYSIS:

Process:

1. **Blood Access:**
   - A vascular access point is created to allow blood to flow from the body to the dialysis machine and back.
   - Common access points include arteriovenous (AV) fistulas, AV grafts, or central venous catheters.
2. **Blood Filtration:**
   - Blood is pumped out of the body and into the dialysis machine, where it passes through a special filter called a dialyzer or artificial kidney.
   - The dialyzer removes waste products, excess fluids, and electrolytes from the blood.
3. **Cleaned Blood Return:**
   - The cleaned blood is then returned to the body.

Frequency:

- Hemodialysis is typically done in sessions, usually three times a week, with each session lasting several hours.

Locations:

- **In-Center Hemodialysis:**
    - Conducted at a dialysis center or hospital.
- **Home Hemodialysis:**
    - Individuals can perform hemodialysis at home, offering more flexibility in scheduling.

2. PERITONEAL DIALYSIS:

Process:

1. **Dialysis Solution:**
    - A sterile dialysis solution (dialysate) is introduced into the peritoneal cavity through a catheter.
    - The peritoneal cavity is the space surrounding the abdominal organs.
2. **Waste Filtration:**
    - The peritoneum acts as a natural filter, allowing waste products and excess fluids to move from the blood vessels into the dialysis solution.
3. **Draining the Solution:**
    - After a dwell time, the used dialysis solution, containing the filtered waste and excess fluids, is drained out of the peritoneal cavity.
4. **Adding Fresh Solution:**
    - Fresh dialysis solution is then introduced for the next cycle.

Frequency:

- Peritoneal dialysis is usually done daily, and it can be performed during the day or overnight.

Locations:

- **Continuous Ambulatory Peritoneal Dialysis (CAPD):**
  - Allows for mobility during the day.
- **Automated Peritoneal Dialysis (APD):**
  - Uses a machine to perform exchanges, often done overnight while the person sleeps.

CONSIDERATIONS FOR BOTH TYPES OF DIALYSIS:

Dietary Restrictions:

- Individuals on dialysis often have dietary restrictions, including limitations on sodium, potassium, phosphorus, and fluid intake.

Medication Management:

- Medications may be prescribed to manage complications associated with kidney failure, such as anemia or bone disease.

Monitoring:

- Regular monitoring of blood levels of electrolytes, waste products, and other markers is essential to assess the effectiveness of the dialysis treatment.

Lifestyle Adjustments:

- Individuals on dialysis may need to make adjustments to their lifestyle, including work schedules, travel plans, and daily activities.

Emotional Support:

- Living with a chronic condition and undergoing regular treatments can have emotional and psychological impacts. Seeking emotional support from friends, family, or support groups is important.

It's crucial for individuals undergoing dialysis to work closely with their healthcare team, including nephrologists and dialysis nurses, to manage their condition effectively. Treatment plans are often individualized based on the specific needs and health status of each patient.

COPING WITH THE CHALLENGES OF REGULAR DIALYSIS

Coping with the challenges of regular dialysis can be a significant aspect of managing kidney failure. The routine of frequent medical appointments, dietary restrictions, and lifestyle adjustments can impact various aspects of life. Here are some strategies to cope with the challenges of regular dialysis:

1. EMOTIONAL SUPPORT:

- **Seek Counseling:** Individual or group counseling can provide a safe space to express feelings, fears, and frustrations associated with kidney failure and dialysis.
- **Support Groups:** Joining a support group for individuals on dialysis can provide a sense of community and understanding. Sharing experiences with others facing similar challenges can be empowering.

2. EDUCATION AND UNDERSTANDING:

- **Learn About Your Condition:** Understanding kidney failure, the dialysis process, and the reasons behind dietary and lifestyle changes can empower you to actively participate in your care.

- **Ask Questions:** Don't hesitate to ask your healthcare team questions. Knowing the purpose and potential outcomes of your treatment can reduce anxiety and uncertainty.

3. ESTABLISH A ROUTINE:

- **Create a Schedule:** Develop a routine that incorporates dialysis sessions, medication schedules, and dietary guidelines. Consistency can help manage stress and create a sense of predictability.
- **Plan Ahead:** Anticipate challenges and plan accordingly. Whether its meal preparation, transportation, or scheduling appointments, having a plan in place can reduce stress.

4. CONNECT WITH OTHERS:

- **Stay Connected:** Maintain connections with friends and family. Social support is crucial during challenging times.
- **Educate Loved Ones:** Help your loved ones understand your condition, treatment, and needs. Their understanding and support can positively impact your emotional well-being.

5. FOCUS ON MENTAL AND PHYSICAL WELL-BEING:

- **Engage in Hobbies:** Pursue activities and hobbies that bring joy and relaxation.
- **Physical Activity:** If your healthcare team approves, engage in regular physical activity suitable for your condition. Exercise can improve mood and overall well-being.

6. NUTRITIONAL SUPPORT:

- **Work with a Dietitian:** Collaborate with a registered dietitian specializing in renal nutrition. They can help create a meal plan that aligns with your dietary restrictions and nutritional needs.

- **Explore Tasty Options:** Experiment with new recipes and flavors within the limits of your dietary restrictions. Finding enjoyable meals can make the process more manageable.

7. ADDRESS FINANCIAL CONCERNS:

- **Financial Counseling:** If you have concerns about the financial aspects of managing kidney failure, consult with a financial counselor. They can provide guidance on available resources and assistance programs.

8. SET REALISTIC GOALS:

- **Celebrate Achievements:** Acknowledge and celebrate small victories along your journey. Setting realistic goals can provide a sense of accomplishment.

9. MAINTAIN OPEN COMMUNICATION:

- **Talk to Your Healthcare Team:** Share your concerns, challenges, and preferences with your healthcare team. They can provide guidance and make adjustments to your treatment plan when necessary.

10. EXPLORE RELAXATION TECHNIQUES:

- **Practice Relaxation:** Techniques such as deep breathing, meditation, or yoga can help manage stress and promote relaxation.

11. CONSIDER MENTAL HEALTH SUPPORT:

- **Therapy or Counseling:** If you're struggling with the emotional impact of kidney failure and dialysis, consider seeking professional mental health support.

12. EXPLORE TRANSPLANT OPTIONS:

- **Discuss Transplantation:** If suitable, discuss the possibility of kidney transplantation with your healthcare team. It may offer a long-term solution and reduce the need for ongoing dialysis.

Coping with regular dialysis involves a holistic approach that addresses physical, emotional, and social well-being. It's essential to tailor coping strategies to your unique needs and circumstances. Regular communication with your healthcare team and the active involvement of supportive friends and family can significantly contribute to your overall coping and adjustment.

CHAPTER SIX
PREVENTING KIDNEY FAILURE

Preventing kidney failure involves adopting a healthy lifestyle and managing risk factors that can contribute to kidney disease. While some factors may be beyond your control, there are several proactive measures you can take to reduce the risk of kidney failure:

LIFESTYLE CHANGES FOR PREVENTION

Adopting a healthy lifestyle is crucial for preventing kidney disease and maintaining overall well-being. Here are lifestyle changes that can contribute to kidney health and reduce the risk of kidney disease:

1. MAINTAIN A BALANCED DIET:

- **Eat a Variety of Foods:** Include a variety of fruits, vegetables, whole grains, and lean proteins in your diet to ensure a well-rounded nutrient intake.
- **Limit Sodium Intake:** Reduce the consumption of high-sodium foods, as excessive sodium can contribute to high blood pressure and kidney damage.

2. STAY HYDRATED:

- **Adequate Fluid Intake:** Drink enough water to stay hydrated. Proper hydration supports kidney function and helps prevent kidney stones.

3. CONTROL BLOOD PRESSURE:

- **Healthy Blood Pressure Levels:** Monitor and manage your blood pressure to keep it within a healthy range. High blood pressure is a major risk factor for kidney disease.

4. MANAGE DIABETES:

- **Blood Sugar Control:** If you have diabetes, manage your blood sugar levels effectively. Uncontrolled diabetes can lead to kidney damage over time.

5. MAINTAIN A HEALTHY WEIGHT:

- **Balanced Diet and Exercise:** Adopt a balanced diet and engage in regular physical activity to achieve and maintain a healthy weight. Obesity is a risk factor for kidney disease.

6. QUIT SMOKING:

- **Smoking Cessation:** If you smoke, quit smoking. Smoking can damage blood vessels and contribute to kidney disease.

7. LIMIT ALCOHOL CONSUMPTION:

- **Moderate Drinking:** If you consume alcohol, do so in moderation. Excessive alcohol intake can have negative effects on kidney health.

8. EXERCISE REGULARLY:

- **Regular Physical Activity:** Incorporate regular exercise into your routine. Exercise helps maintain a healthy weight, control blood pressure, and improve overall cardiovascular health.

9. MANAGE STRESS:

- **Stress Reduction Techniques:** Practice stress reduction techniques such as deep breathing, meditation, yoga, or other activities that promote relaxation.

10. LIMIT OVER-THE-COUNTER MEDICATIONS:

- **Safe Medication Use:** Use over-the-counter medications, including pain relievers, as directed. Some medications can cause kidney damage if used excessively.

11. REGULAR HEALTH CHECK-UPS:

- **Routine Medical Exams:** Attend regular check-ups with your healthcare provider. Include kidney function tests in routine health screenings, especially if you have risk factors for kidney disease.

12. LIMIT PHOSPHORUS INTAKE:

- **Phosphorus Awareness:** If you have kidney disease, limit phosphorus intake. High phosphorus levels can contribute to bone and heart problems.

13. AVOID NEPHROTOXIC SUBSTANCES:

- **Be Cautious with Certain Substances:** Limit exposure to substances that can be harmful to the kidneys, including certain medications, environmental toxins, and excessive use of pain relievers.

14. GET ADEQUATE SLEEP:

- **Quality Sleep:** Ensure you get enough quality sleep each night. Poor sleep can contribute to various health issues, including kidney problems.

15. STAY INFORMED:

- **Educate Yourself:** Learn about kidney health, risk factors for kidney disease, and lifestyle measures to protect your kidneys.

16. FAMILY HISTORY AWARENESS:

- **Family Health History:** Be aware of your family's health history, especially regarding kidney disease. If there's a family history, discuss it with your healthcare provider for appropriate monitoring.

17. LIMIT RED MEAT CONSUMPTION:

- **Moderate Red Meat Intake:** Limit the consumption of red meat, especially processed meats. High intake may be associated with an increased risk of kidney disease.

18. MODERATE PROTEIN INTAKE:

- **Balanced Protein Consumption:** While protein is essential, excessive protein intake, especially from animal sources, may strain the kidneys. Consume protein in moderation.

19. AVOID EXCESSIVE USE OF NSAIDS:

- **Safe Pain Management:** Limit the use of nonsteroidal anti-inflammatory drugs (NSAIDs) as they can contribute to kidney damage if used excessively.

Adopting these lifestyle changes can contribute significantly to kidney health and reduce the risk of kidney disease. It's important to consult with your healthcare provider before making significant changes to your lifestyle, especially if you have existing health conditions. Regular medical check-ups and proactive management of risk factors are essential for maintaining kidney health over the long term.

MANAGING CHRONIC CONDITIONS

Managing chronic conditions is essential for overall health and well-being, and it becomes particularly crucial when aiming to prevent kidney disease. Here are strategies for effectively managing common chronic conditions that can impact kidney health:

1. HYPERTENSION (HIGH BLOOD PRESSURE):

- **Medication Adherence:** Take blood pressure medications as prescribed by your healthcare provider. Adhering to the prescribed medication regimen is crucial for controlling hypertension.
- **Regular Monitoring:** Keep track of your blood pressure at home and attend regular check-ups with your healthcare provider for monitoring and adjustments.

2. DIABETES:

- **Blood Sugar Control:** Manage your blood sugar levels effectively through medication, lifestyle changes, and regular monitoring.
- **Healthy Diet:** Adopt a balanced and low-glycemic diet. Consult with a registered dietitian for personalized dietary guidance.
- **Regular Exercise:** Engage in regular physical activity, as it can help improve insulin sensitivity and overall diabetes management.

3. CHRONIC KIDNEY DISEASE (CKD):

- **Follow Treatment Plan:** If you already have chronic kidney disease, follow your healthcare provider's treatment plan, including medications, dietary restrictions, and lifestyle modifications.
- **Regular Monitoring:** Attend regular check-ups to monitor kidney function, blood pressure, and other relevant markers.
- **Dietary Modifications:** Work with a dietitian to create a kidney-friendly diet tailored to your specific needs and stage of kidney disease.

4. HEART DISEASE:

- **Medication Adherence:** If you have heart disease, take prescribed medications regularly to manage your condition.

- **Healthy Lifestyle:** Adopt heart-healthy habits, including a balanced diet, regular exercise, smoking cessation, and stress management.

5. OBESITY:

- **Weight Management:** If overweight, work towards achieving and maintaining a healthy weight through a combination of a balanced diet and regular physical activity.
- **Consult a Specialist:** Consider consulting with a healthcare professional, such as a dietitian or a fitness expert, for personalized guidance.

6. DYSLIPIDEMIA (HIGH CHOLESTEROL):

- **Medication Adherence:** Take prescribed cholesterol-lowering medications as directed by your healthcare provider.
- **Heart-Healthy Diet:** Adopt a diet low in saturated and trans fats. Include heart-healthy fats from sources like olive oil and fatty fish.

7. AUTOIMMUNE DISORDERS:

- **Medication Management:** Adhere to prescribed medications for autoimmune disorders as directed by your healthcare provider.
- **Regular Monitoring:** Attend regular check-ups to monitor the progression of the autoimmune condition and its potential impact on kidney health.

8. THYROID DISORDERS:

- **Medication Adherence:** If you have a thyroid disorder, take thyroid medications as prescribed.
- **Regular Thyroid Monitoring:** Attend regular thyroid function tests to ensure appropriate medication dosages.

9. RESPIRATORY CONDITIONS (E.G., COPD, ASTHMA):

- **Medication Adherence:** Take prescribed medications for respiratory conditions as directed.
- **Lifestyle Adjustments:** Manage triggers and adopt a healthy lifestyle to support respiratory health.

10. GASTROINTESTINAL CONDITIONS:

- **Medication Adherence:** Take medications as prescribed for gastrointestinal conditions.
- **Dietary Modifications:** Make dietary adjustments to manage symptoms and support overall digestive health.

11. CHRONIC PAIN CONDITIONS:

- **Pain Management Plan:** Work with your healthcare provider to develop a comprehensive pain management plan that may include medications, physical therapy, and lifestyle modifications.
- **Balanced Approach:** Strive for a balance between pain management and avoiding activities that may exacerbate the condition.

12. NEUROLOGICAL CONDITIONS:

- **Medication Adherence:** Take medications as prescribed for neurological conditions.
- **Regular Follow-ups:** Attend regular follow-ups with neurologists or specialists overseeing your condition.

13. MENTAL HEALTH CONDITIONS:

- **Therapeutic Support:** Seek mental health support through counseling, therapy, or psychiatric care.
- **Medication Management:** If prescribed medications for mental health conditions, take them as directed.

14. REGULAR HEALTH CHECK-UPS:

- **Comprehensive Health Monitoring:** Attend regular check-ups with your primary care provider to monitor overall health and address emerging concerns promptly.

15. LIFESTYLE MODIFICATIONS:

- **Healthy Lifestyle Habits:** Adopt a healthy lifestyle, including regular exercise, a balanced diet, adequate sleep, and stress management.

16. MEDICATION REVIEW:

- **Regular Medication Review:** Periodically review medications with your healthcare provider to assess their effectiveness and make adjustments as needed.

17. PATIENT EDUCATION:

- **Stay Informed:** Educate yourself about your chronic conditions, treatment options, and lifestyle modifications. Informed patients are better equipped to manage their health.

18. COLLABORATE WITH HEALTHCARE PROVIDERS:

- **Open Communication:** Maintain open communication with your healthcare providers. Share any concerns, changes in symptoms, or challenges you may be facing.

19. SUPPORT SYSTEM:

- **Build a Support System:** Surround yourself with a supportive network of family, friends, and healthcare professionals who can assist and encourage you on your health journey.

Effective management of chronic conditions requires a collaborative approach between patients and healthcare providers. Regular communication, adherence to treatment plans, and proactive lifestyle modifications are key components of successful chronic disease management. Always consult with your healthcare team for personalized advice based on your unique health needs and conditions.

REGULAR HEALTH CHECKUPS

Regular health checkups are essential for maintaining overall well-being, preventing diseases, and detecting health issues early when they are more manageable. The frequency and specific components of checkups may vary based on age, gender, medical history, and individual risk factors. Here are some general guidelines for regular health checkups:

1. ANNUAL CHECKUPS:

- **Primary Care Visit:** Schedule an annual visit with your primary care provider (PCP). This allows for a comprehensive assessment of your overall health.
- **Blood Pressure Monitoring:** Regularly monitor your blood pressure, and have it checked during your annual visit.

2. BIENNIAL OR PERIODIC CHECKUPS:

- **Dental Checkups:** Visit the dentist for routine cleanings and checkups every six months to a year, or as recommended by your dentist.
- **Vision Exams:** Have your eyes checked every 1-2 years, or more often if you wear glasses or contact lenses.
- **Skin Exams:** Periodically check your skin for changes in moles or unusual spots. See a dermatologist if you notice anything concerning.

3. SCREENINGS BASED ON AGE AND RISK FACTORS:

- **Cholesterol Testing:** Starting in your 20s, regular cholesterol screenings may be recommended, especially if you have risk factors for heart disease.
- **Blood Sugar Testing:** Consider regular blood sugar testing, especially if you have diabetes risk factors.
- **Cancer Screenings:** Follow recommended cancer screenings based on age, gender, and family history. This may include mammograms, Pap smears, prostate exams, colonoscopies, and more.
- **Bone Density Testing:** For postmenopausal women and older adults, bone density testing may be recommended to assess osteoporosis risk.

4. IMMUNIZATIONS:

- **Vaccinations:** Stay up-to-date with vaccinations as recommended by your healthcare provider. This may include flu shots, tetanus boosters, pneumonia vaccines, and others.

5. MENTAL HEALTH CHECKUPS:

- **Psychological Assessments:** Consider periodic mental health checkups, especially if you have a history of mental health conditions. Discuss any concerns or changes in mood with your healthcare provider.
- **Therapy or Counseling:** If needed, engage in therapy or counseling sessions to address mental health concerns.

6. REPRODUCTIVE HEALTH:

- **Gynecological Exams:** Women should have regular gynecological exams, including Pap smears and screenings for sexually transmitted infections.
- **Prostate Exams:** Men, especially those with a family history or other risk factors, may need periodic prostate exams.

7. MEDICAL IMAGING:

- **X-rays, MRIs, CT Scans:** Medical imaging may be recommended based on specific health concerns or symptoms. Examples include X-rays for bone injuries, MRIs for soft tissue evaluation, or CT scans for certain conditions.

8. BLOOD TESTS:

- **Routine Blood Tests:** Periodic blood tests can assess various health markers, including blood cell counts, kidney function, liver function, and more.

9. WEIGHT AND BMI MONITORING:

- **Regular Weight Check:** Keep track of your weight and body mass index (BMI) to monitor changes over time.

10. DIET AND NUTRITION REVIEW:

- **Nutritional Assessment:** Discuss your diet and nutrition with your healthcare provider. They can provide guidance on maintaining a healthy diet.

11. EXERCISE AND PHYSICAL ACTIVITY:

- **Physical Activity Assessment:** Discuss your exercise routine with your healthcare provider and assess whether it aligns with recommended levels of physical activity.

12. MEDICATION REVIEW:

- **Medication Management:** Regularly review your medications with your healthcare provider. Ensure that dosages are appropriate, and discuss any side effects or concerns.

13. FAMILY HEALTH HISTORY REVIEW:

- **Update Health History:** Periodically update your healthcare provider on any changes in your family health history. This information can be crucial for assessing your risk factors.

14. LIFESTYLE COUNSELING:

- **Health Promotion Counseling:** Receive guidance on healthy lifestyle choices, including smoking cessation, alcohol moderation, stress management, and more.

15. Blood Donation:

- **Donate Blood:** If eligible, consider donating blood regularly. This not only supports community health but also allows for routine health checks on certain markers.

16. VISION AND HEARING CHECKS:

- **Vision and Hearing Tests:** Periodically have your vision and hearing tested, especially as you age.

Regular health checkups are an integral part of preventive healthcare. They facilitate early detection of potential health issues, allow for timely intervention, and contribute to the maintenance of good health. It's important to communicate openly with your healthcare provider about any concerns, changes in your health, or new symptoms you may be experiencing.

CHAPTER SEVEN
LIVING WITH A TRANSPLANTED KIDNEY

Living with a transplanted kidney is a transformative experience that can significantly improve quality of life for individuals who have undergone kidney transplantation. Here are key aspects of life after kidney transplantation:

THE TRANSPLANT PROCESS

The transplant process is a complex and highly coordinated series of events that involves various healthcare professionals, thorough evaluations, and careful planning. Here is an overview of the key steps in the kidney transplant process:

1. REFERRAL AND EVALUATION:

- **Referral:** The process often begins with a referral from a nephrologist (kidney specialist) or another healthcare provider who identifies a patient as a potential candidate for kidney transplantation.
- **Initial Evaluation:** The transplant team conducts an initial evaluation to assess the patient's overall health, medical history, and suitability for transplantation.

2. COMPREHENSIVE MEDICAL AND PSYCHOSOCIAL ASSESSMENTS:

- **Medical Tests:** A series of medical tests are conducted to assess kidney function, blood type, tissue compatibility, and overall health. This includes blood tests, imaging studies, and other diagnostic procedures.

- **Psychosocial Evaluation:** A thorough psychosocial assessment is performed to evaluate the patient's mental health, social support system, and ability to adhere to post-transplant care requirements.

3. PATIENT EDUCATION:

- **Educational Sessions:** Transplant candidates and their families undergo education sessions to understand the transplant process, potential risks, benefits, and the importance of adherence to medications and lifestyle changes.

4. LISTING ON THE TRANSPLANT WAITLIST:

- **Matched with a Donor:** If a living donor is available, the transplant surgery can be scheduled. If not, the patient is placed on the national transplant waiting list to receive a deceased donor kidney.
- **Organ Procurement and Transplantation Network (OPTN):** The United Network for Organ Sharing (UNOS) manages the OPTN, a national database that matches donors with recipients based on compatibility.

5. LIVING DONOR EVALUATION (IF APPLICABLE):

- **Donor Evaluation:** If the patient has a living donor, the donor undergoes a thorough evaluation process to ensure compatibility and assess the donor's overall health and willingness to donate.

6. PRE-TRANSPLANT SURGERY EVALUATION:

- **Final Health Assessment:** As the scheduled transplant date approaches, the patient undergoes a final health assessment to ensure that they are still suitable for surgery.

7. TRANSPLANT SURGERY:

- **Recipient Surgery:** The recipient undergoes kidney transplant surgery, during which the donated kidney is implanted.
- **Donor Surgery (if living donor):** The living donor undergoes surgery to remove a kidney for transplantation.

8. POST-TRANSPLANT CARE:

- **Monitoring:** The recipient is closely monitored in the immediate post-transplant period in the hospital to ensure the new kidney functions properly and to manage any complications.
- **Medication Regimen:** The patient is prescribed a regimen of immunosuppressive medications to prevent rejection of the transplanted organ. Other medications may also be prescribed to manage potential side effects and prevent infections.

9. RECOVERY AND REHABILITATION:

- **Hospital Stay:** The length of the hospital stay varies, but most patients are discharged within a week after surgery.
- **Follow-up Visits:** The patient has regular follow-up visits with the transplant team to monitor kidney function, adjust medications, and address any concerns.

10. LONG-TERM MANAGEMENT:

- **Medication Adherence:** Lifelong adherence to prescribed medications, particularly immunosuppressants, is crucial to prevent rejection.
- **Regular Monitoring:** Regular follow-up appointments, blood tests, and imaging studies are scheduled to monitor kidney function and overall health.

11. LIVING WITH A TRANSPLANTED KIDNEY:

- **Return to Normal Activities:** Once cleared by the healthcare team, recipients can often return to normal activities, including work, travel, and recreational pursuits.
- **Lifestyle Adjustments:** Recipients may need to make certain lifestyle adjustments, including dietary modifications and regular exercise, to maintain overall health.

12. GRATITUDE AND REFLECTION:

- **Expressing Gratitude:** Many transplant recipients express gratitude for the gift of life from the donor and their family. Some recipients choose to connect with the donor family, while others prefer to remain anonymous.

13. SUPPORT SYSTEMS:

- **Psychosocial Support:** Ongoing psychosocial support, including counseling and support groups, can be beneficial for both transplant recipients and living donors.

14. LONG-TERM FOLLOW-UP:

- **Lifelong Monitoring:** Transplant recipients require lifelong monitoring to ensure the ongoing success of the transplant and address any emerging health issues.

The transplant process is a collaborative effort involving transplant surgeons, nephrologists, transplant coordinators, social workers, and other healthcare professionals. Communication and collaboration between the patient and the healthcare team are crucial for a successful transplant journey.

POST-TRANSPLANT CARE

Post-transplant care is a critical phase in the kidney transplant journey, and it involves ongoing medical monitoring, adherence to medications, lifestyle adjustments, and regular follow-up appointments. Here are key aspects of post-transplant care:

1. MEDICATION ADHERENCE:

- **Immunosuppressive Medications:** Take immunosuppressive medications as prescribed without missing doses. These medications are essential to prevent rejection of the transplanted kidney.
- **Follow Medication Schedule:** Adhere to the prescribed medication schedule, including the timing and dosage instructions provided by the transplant team.
- **Communicate Changes:** Inform the transplant team about any changes in medications, including over-the-counter drugs, supplements, or herbal remedies.

2. REGULAR MONITORING:

- **Blood Tests:** Undergo regular blood tests to monitor kidney function, medication levels, and overall health.
- **Imaging Studies:** Periodically, imaging studies such as ultrasounds or biopsies may be performed to assess the health of the transplanted kidney.

3. DIET AND NUTRITION:

- **Balanced Diet:** Maintain a balanced and healthy diet. Consult with a dietitian to address any dietary restrictions and ensure proper nutrition.
- **Hydration:** Stay adequately hydrated. However, follow any fluid restrictions recommended by the transplant team.

4. LIFESTYLE ADJUSTMENTS:

- **Exercise:** Engage in regular, moderate exercise to promote overall health. Discuss with the transplant team before starting a new exercise routine.
- **Avoid Smoking:** If you smoke, quit smoking. Smoking can have adverse effects on both the transplanted kidney and overall health.
- **Limit Alcohol:** Consume alcohol in moderation. Discuss alcohol limits with the transplant team.

5. INFECTION PREVENTION:

- **Hygiene Practices:** Practice good hygiene to reduce the risk of infections. Wash hands regularly and avoid contact with sick individuals.
- **Vaccinations:** Stay up-to-date on vaccinations as recommended by the transplant team. Certain vaccinations may be contraindicated, so consult before getting any immunizations.

6. REGULAR FOLLOW-UP APPOINTMENTS:

- **Transplant Clinic Visits:** Attend regular follow-up appointments with the transplant clinic. These visits are crucial for monitoring kidney function, adjusting medications, and addressing any concerns.
- **Screening for Complications:** Regular check-ups allow the healthcare team to screen for potential complications and address them promptly.

7. MONITORING FOR REJECTION:

- **Know the Signs:** Be aware of signs of rejection, such as changes in urine output, swelling, weight gain, or flu-like symptoms. Report any concerning symptoms to the transplant team immediately.
- **Biopsy (if needed):** In some cases, a kidney biopsy may be performed to assess the health of the transplanted kidney tissue.

8. PSYCHOSOCIAL SUPPORT:

- **Counseling and Support Groups:** Consider participating in counseling or support groups to address any emotional or psychological challenges related to the transplant experience.
- **Expressing Gratitude:** Many transplant recipients find gratitude and reflection helpful in their emotional well-being.

9. FAMILY PLANNING:

- **Discuss With Healthcare Team:** If family planning is a consideration, discuss it with the transplant team. Certain medications may need to be adjusted during pregnancy.

10. MEDICATION REVIEW:

- **Regular Medication Review:** Periodically review medications with the transplant team. Adjustments may be made based on kidney function, side effects, and overall health.

11. FINANCIAL CONSIDERATIONS:

- **Insurance Coverage:** Ensure that you have appropriate insurance coverage for post-transplant care, medications, and potential complications.
- **Financial Counseling:** Consult with a financial counselor to address any financial concerns related to ongoing healthcare costs.

12. LIVING A FULL LIFE:

- **Resume Normal Activities:** Once cleared by the healthcare team, resume normal activities, including work, travel, and recreational pursuits.
- **Pursue Passions:** Embrace opportunities to pursue personal and professional goals, knowing that the transplanted kidney has provided a new lease on life.

13. LONG-TERM MONITORING:

- **Lifelong Monitoring:** Continue with lifelong monitoring to ensure the ongoing success of the transplant and address any emerging health issues.

14. SUPPORT SYSTEMS:

- **Maintain Support Networks:** Surround yourself with supportive friends, family, and healthcare professionals who can assist and encourage you on your post-transplant journey.

15. EDUCATION AND AWARENESS:

- **Stay Informed:** Educate yourself about post-transplant care, potential risks, and how to care for your transplanted kidney. Knowledge empowers you to actively participate in your health.

16. PATIENT ADVOCACY:

- **Advocate for Yourself:** Be an advocate for your health. Communicate openly with the transplant team, ask questions, and actively participate in decisions related to your care.

Post-transplant care is a lifelong commitment, and success depends on your active involvement in managing your health. Regular communication with the transplant team, adherence to medical recommendations, and a focus on overall well-being contribute to a successful and fulfilling life with a transplanted kidney.

EMOTIONAL AND PHYSICAL RECOVERY

Emotional and physical recovery after kidney transplantation is a multifaceted process that requires time, support, and active participation from both the transplant recipient and their support network. Here's a breakdown of the emotional and physical aspects of recovery:

EMOTIONAL RECOVERY:

1. **EXPECT A RANGE OF EMOTIONS:**
   - **Gratitude:** Many transplant recipients experience profound gratitude for the gift of life and the opportunity for improved health.
   - **Anxiety and Fear:** It's normal to feel anxious or fearful about the success of the transplant and potential complications.
   - **Relief:** Relief from the burdens of dialysis and the anticipation of improved health are common emotions.
2. **COUNSELING AND SUPPORT GROUPS:**
   - **Psychological Support:** Engage in counseling or join support groups to address the emotional challenges associated with transplantation.
   - **Peer Support:** Connect with other transplant recipients who can share their experiences and offer valuable insights.
3. **EXPRESSING GRATITUDE:**
   - **Acknowledging Donor Families:** Some recipients find solace and closure by expressing gratitude to the donor's family through anonymous letters or facilitated communication.
4. **DEALING WITH GRIEF AND LOSS:**
   - **Acknowledging Loss:** While transplantation is a life-saving procedure, it's essential to acknowledge any grief or loss associated with the transplant journey.
5. **MENTAL HEALTH CARE:**
   - **Regular Check-ins:** Schedule regular check-ins with mental health professionals to address any emerging concerns.
   - **Mindfulness and Relaxation Techniques:** Practice mindfulness, meditation, or relaxation techniques to manage stress and promote emotional well-being.

PHYSICAL RECOVERY:

1. **POST-SURGERY HEALING:**
   - **Hospital Stay:** The initial recovery period occurs in the hospital, where medical professionals monitor vital signs, manage pain, and ensure the proper functioning of the transplanted kidney.
   - **Follow Care Instructions:** Follow post-surgery care instructions, including wound care and medication management.
2. **MEDICATION ADHERENCE:**
   - **Immunosuppressive Medications:** Take immunosuppressive medications as prescribed to prevent rejection. Adhering to the medication regimen is crucial for long-term success.
   - **Side Effect Management:** Work closely with the healthcare team to manage any medication-related side effects.
3. **GRADUAL RETURN TO NORMAL ACTIVITIES:**
   - **Mobility:** Gradually reintroduce physical activities, starting with gentle movements and progressing as advised by the healthcare team.
   - **Resume Daily Life:** As recovery progresses, resume daily activities, such as walking, cooking, and light chores.
4. **EXERCISE AND REHABILITATION:**
   - **Structured Exercise Program:** Engage in a structured exercise program, incorporating both aerobic activities and strength training, as approved by the healthcare team.
   - **Physical Therapy:** If needed, participate in physical therapy to aid in recovery and improve strength and mobility.
5. **NUTRITION AND DIETARY GUIDELINES:**
   - **Balanced Diet:** Follow dietary guidelines provided by a dietitian to ensure proper nutrition and support overall health.
   - **Fluid Intake:** Monitor fluid intake as per recommendations, taking into account any specific restrictions.

6. **REGULAR CHECK-UPS AND MONITORING:**
   - **Follow-up Appointments:** Attend regular follow-up appointments with the transplant team to monitor kidney function, adjust medications, and address any concerns.
   - **Blood Tests and Imaging:** Undergo periodic blood tests and imaging studies to assess the health of the transplanted kidney.
7. **INFECTION PREVENTION:**
   - **Hygiene Practices:** Practice good hygiene to prevent infections. Follow the transplant team's recommendations for avoiding potential sources of infection.
   - **Vaccinations:** Stay up-to-date on vaccinations as recommended by the transplant team.
8. **COMMUNICATION WITH HEALTHCARE TEAM:**
   - **Open Communication:** Maintain open and honest communication with the healthcare team. Report any changes in health, medications, or concerns promptly.
9. **REHABILITATION FOR LIVING DONORS (IF APPLICABLE):**
   - **Living Donor Recovery:** If a living donor is involved, they will also undergo a recovery process. Support and open communication between donors and recipients are essential.
10. **RETURNING TO WORK AND NORMAL ROUTINE:**
    - **Consult with Healthcare Team:** Before returning to work or resuming normal routines, consult with the healthcare team to ensure it aligns with your recovery progress.
11. **SEXUAL HEALTH:**
    - **Consult with Healthcare Team:** If you have concerns about sexual health, discuss them with the healthcare team. They can provide guidance and address any potential issues.
12. **MONITORING AND ADDRESSING COMPLICATIONS:**
    - **Vigilance for Complications:** Be vigilant for any signs of complications, such as rejection, infection, or side effects from medications. Promptly report any concerns to the healthcare team.

Emotional and physical recovery is a gradual process, and the pace varies for each individual. Both aspects are interconnected, with emotional well-being influencing physical health and vice versa. It's crucial to follow the guidance of the transplant team, engage in open communication, and actively participate in the recovery process to ensure the best possible outcomes.

CHAPTER EIGHT
CONCLUSION

In conclusion, the journey through kidney failure, transplantation, and recovery is a profound and transformative experience that encompasses physical, emotional, and lifestyle dimensions. Throughout this process, individuals and their support networks navigate challenges, make crucial decisions, and demonstrate remarkable resilience. From understanding the causes and risk factors of kidney failure to exploring treatment options, lifestyle changes, and the emotional impact, the comprehensive nature of managing kidney health requires a holistic approach.

The medical perspectives, including the diagnosis and treatment of kidney failure, highlight the importance of early detection, accurate diagnosis, and personalized care plans. Advances in medical science, including medications, dialysis, and transplantation, offer hope and improved outcomes for those facing kidney-related challenges.

The emotional and psychological impact of kidney failure and transplantation cannot be overstated. Coping with the diagnosis, navigating the emotional rollercoaster, and building strong support systems are integral components of the journey. Emotional recovery, intertwined with physical well-being, underscores the importance of mental health care, counseling, and open communication with healthcare providers.

The significance of lifestyle changes for kidney health, including diet and nutrition, exercise, and overall well-being, cannot be overstressed. Creating and maintaining a kidney-friendly lifestyle plays a vital role in managing the condition and promoting long-term health.

Living with a transplanted kidney opens a new chapter marked by gratitude, resilience, and the pursuit of a fulfilling life. Post-transplant care, including medication adherence, regular monitoring, and a commitment to a healthy lifestyle, is essential for the long-term success of the transplant.

Inspiring stories of resilience from individuals who have faced kidney-related challenges serve as beacons of hope, demonstrating the transformative power of the human spirit in overcoming adversity.

In essence, the conclusion is an acknowledgment of the complex and multifaceted nature of kidney health, emphasizing the importance of a comprehensive and collaborative approach that involves medical professionals, individuals, and their support networks. It is a call to action for continued awareness, research, and advocacy to improve kidney health outcomes and enhance the quality of life for those affected by kidney disease.